I0426608

THE MYTH THAT KILLS

THE SILENT KILLER THAT NO ONE TELLS US ABOUT

BY WALTER T. JONES

© Copyright 2006 Walter T. Jones.
All rights reserved. No part of this publication may be reproduced, stored in a retrieval system, or transmitted, in any form or by any means, electronic, mechanical, photocopying, recording, or otherwise, without the written prior permission of the author.

Note for Librarians: A cataloguing record for this book is available from Library and Archives Canada at www.collectionscanada.ca/amicus/index-e.html
ISBN 1-4120-8999-9

Printed on paper with minimum 30% recycled fibre.
Trafford's print shop runs on "green energy" from solar, wind and other environmentally-friendly power sources.

TRAFFORD
PUBLISHING™
Offices in Canada, USA, Ireland and UK

Book sales for North America and international:
Trafford Publishing, 6E–2333 Government St.,
Victoria, BC V8T 4P4 CANADA
phone 250 383 6864 (toll-free 1 888 232 4444)
fax 250 383 6804; email to orders@trafford.com
Book sales in Europe:
Trafford Publishing (UK) Limited, 9 Park End Street, 2nd Floor
Oxford, UK OX1 1HH UNITED KINGDOM
phone 44 (0)1865 722 113 (local rate 0845 230 9601)
facsimile 44 (0)1865 722 868; info.uk@trafford.com
Order online at:
trafford.com/06-0755

10 9 8 7 6 5 4 3

Preface

While staying with my Daughter and her family in Florida, I noticed when I woke up every morning, that I felt lousy, drowsy and very tired. Well…

I have lived in a lot of apartments, a lot of hotels and a lot of motels over the years and everywhere that I lived I would always have a window open and/or usually kept the front door open for two reasons. First I always liked the fresh air and second I almost all the time had people coming and going so it was easier to just leave the door open rather than having to get up all the time to open it.

Well, I remembered that when I was up in the High Sierras in California, I used to love the smell of the fresh air. It felt so good to take a breath of the mountain air because it is always so fresh and clean. When I remembered this I thought I would open a window or a door to get some fresh air in the house. In the back door there was a "glass louvered" window so I thought that I would just open the louvers with the crank that is usually on the door and allow some fresh air to come in. Well… when I looked for the crank it was gone. So… I thought that I could just pull on the louvers and they would open. **Not true !**

The louvers had been glued shut with silicone cement. I could not believe my eyes! Why would anyone do such a ridicules thing ? And then I also noticed that the door and windows had all been sealed with weather stripping to keep the outside air from coming in.

I could not believe this so I commented to my Daughter's boyfriend and he immediately started talking about the cost of his electric bill and the fact that leaving the doors and/or windows open would make his electric bill go sky high. Well — his electric bill is already "sky high" and I proved to him that leaving his windows and/or doors open would not make a significant difference and even if it cost a couple of dollars a month more, it is worth it. AND I proved to him that he should have cross ventilation in his house in order to have healthy clean air to breath for him and his family. This was a very difficult thing for him to believe due to the fact that he (and so many others) have been programmed since childhood to — **"KEEP THE DOORS CLOSED"** — **"TURN OFF THE LIGHTS"** — **"CLOSE THE WINDOWS"** —

"TURN DOWN THE THERMOSTAT" — "BLA-BLA-BLA." These instructions are drilled into our heads from childhood by "well meaning parents," "well meaning" relatives, friends and neighbors. **"AND THE AIR CONDITIONING COMPANIES"** and some Agencies. **THESE ARE WRONG!**

Well, to prove my point I went on the Internet and did some research and here is what I found:

With the abundance of reports that I located on the Internet, I proved that this most commonly believed **"MYTH"** is not only false but... **It is KILLING PEOPLE here in this country and also around the World.**

Copywrite©2006TransWorld International

Some of the State Agencies and almost all of the "Air Conditioning" companies make claims that weatherizing your house, apartment and/or buildings will conserve electricity (and/or other energy sources) and save you a lot of money on your heating and air conditioning bills. They claim that the average savings is about $57 dollars a year. I figure that this amounts to about 10 cents a day or $2 or $3 dollars a month.

Is it really worth that small saving to jeopardize your health and the health of your family and your loved ones? NO — it is NOT!

Right away my Daughter wanted to believe it because of course I am her father but mainly because she likes fresh air too and the fact that she could tell the difference when we let in some fresh air. As soon as we started keeping some of the windows and doors open once in awhile, we all started feeling a lot better.

WHAT THESE COMPANIES AND PEOPLE DON'T TELL YOU

They don't tell you is this. <u>**Over four million people die each year in this country alone**</u> **from illnesses related to "Indoor Air Pollution" mainly from keeping windows and doors closed all the time.**

You will see the proof and some very interesting details in this report. The things in this report are to enlighten you and show you the truth about —

<u>**"THE MYTH THAT KILLS"**</u>

and — how you can help improve AND PROTECT your health and the health of your family — especially your young children. AND...

"THE FREE CURE"

You will also learn in this book about "THE FREE CURE" and how simple it is for you and your family to utilize, so that you may start using it immediately.

CONCLUSION

What really made me happy is this: the fact that I was able to find plenty of reports on the Internet that **verified that what I had been saying was in fact true** and in this book you will find many reports along with the URL's — Internet addresses — so that you may verify these facts yourself and prove that this **"TRADITIONAL MYTH" IS REALLY TOTALLY FALSE. AND...**

What also makes me happy is the fact that I am able to help you avoid this unhealthy "FALSE MYTH" and show you the "FREE CURE" so that you may help protect your health and the health of your family.

SPREAD THE WORD AND HELP YOUR FRIENDS, YOUR RELATIVES AND YOUR NEIGHBORS PROTECT THEIR HEALTH AND THE HEALTH OF THEIR LOVED ONES.

Walter T. Jones

About the Author

The author of this book Mr. Walter T. Jones is more than highly qualified to have done the research and investigation that went into compiling the facts in this book.

His credentials are as follows:

Mr. Jones is retired from McDonnell Aircraft as a Senior Engineer Scientist and has had the honor to serve as a consulting Engineer for the following US Companies.

In the mid 1960's he worked for Librascope Inc. a division of General Precision in Burbank California supervising the manufacture of the 473L Data Processing System for the US Air Force's ANFQY-11 World Wide Communication Program for the Pentagon in Washington DC which unknowingly (at that time) was the beginning of the Internet that we know today.

After conducting this huge project Jones went on to work for such companies as; Lockheed Aircraft (L-1011 Tri-Star), Hughes Aircraft, Hughes Electro-Optical (Satellites), Northrop Aircraft (F-18, F-20, F-5 Etc.), McDonnell Douglas Aircraft (T-45, MD-11, MD80-90 Etc.), Aero-Jet General (Photo-Plane for Global-GSM Satellite tracking systems), Litton Industries (Inertia Guidance Systems), Dupont Instrument Division (Mass Spectrometers), Ana Tronics Corporation (Automated Blood Analyzers for Hospitals), Space General (Re-Entry Systems for Spacecraft) and more.

He is a qualified efficiency specialist, problem solver, concept design engineer for new designs and redesigns and research engineer.

He suggests that when reading this book that you put your customs and traditional beliefs aside and approach these most important facts with an open mind. Don't let prior teachings interfere with your thoughts and pre-occupied thoughts sway your thinking and your judgment.

While you were probably taught (by well meaning parents, well meaning friends, family members and neighbors), that the proper thing to do is to keep doors and windows closed in order to conserve electricity, it will be proven to you in this book that this is the wrong thing to do in order to protect your health and the health of your children and your loved ones.

And — It could possibly save your life.

It is his hope and desire that the information in this book will help save the lives of those who could possibly die from some of the illnesses and diseases related to **"INDOOR AIR POLLUTION"** and also help protect the health of some of those who might become affected by some of the illnesses and diseases related to "INDOOR AIR POLLUTION" — before it is too late, for those unaware and those who have not been properly warned.

The general public is never even told or warned about the devastating results that Indoor air pollution can cause and do cause. 3.6 MILLION PEOPLE DIE EACH YEAR in this country alone and there are more that die each year in other countries.

* * * * *

There are essentials for Life that include Food, Water, Rest and of course The Air We Breath — **BUT... for good health —**

FRESH CLEAN AIR IS A <u>MUST</u>!

To those who have died needlessly and to their loved ones who know now that their tragedy could have been prevented if only they had been warned.

I truly wish that I had written this book sooner. Some of these people could have been saved and some of you might have not suffered your losses.

WT Jones

The Myth That Kills
BY WALTER T JONES

* * * * *

This is a report based on many years of research and taken from various reports collected from City Government agencies, Medical Reports from Doctors and Scientists, information from Web MD and many other bonified sources.
The sources are listed in this book with URL addresses.

* * * * *

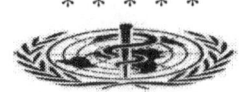

HEALTH WATCH

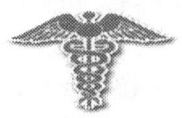

— Medical Alert —
Save a Life — It may be your own

The Myth That Kills - That Nobody Tells Us About

THE MYTH THAT KILLS
The — SILENT KILLER THAT...

"NO ONE TELLS US ABOUT"

— THIS REPORT WILL SURPRISE YOU —

You may be at risk and your children and your loved ones may also be at risk! We are led to believe that our homes are a safe place to be?

Not true!

Every Home Is At Risk — Just Wait 'Til You See Why!
THE SECRET IS OUT!

MILLIONS OF UNSUSPECTING PEOPLE HAVE DIED
(— ESTIMATED 3.6 Million DIE each year —)

and it's a shame because now... it is too late for them.
BUT... For You... It's not too late... THE SECRET IS OUT!

* * * * *

A FREE CURE? YES! AND IT IS VERY SIMPLE!

9

THE MYTH THAT KILLS THAT NOBODY TELLS US ABOUT

HOW COULD 250 MILLION PEOPLE BE SO WRONG?

I'LL TELL YOU HOW!

People in this country are wrong!

And people in a lot of other countries are wrong also!

WHAT YOU REALLY NEED TO KNOW...

(GET FREE INFO NOW)
REFER TO INTERNET SITES (URLs)
LISTED ON FOLLOWING PAGES

* * * * *

FREE CURE? YES!

THE SECRET IS OUT! READ THIS!

* * * * *

All homes should be tested for RADON GAS regardless of geographic location. It costs only about $10 bucks on the Internet.
REF.
Quote from:
Compiled by Jim Brueggemeyer,
Industrial Hygiene Technician
Kimbrough Ambulatory Care Center,
Fort George G. Meade, Md.

All of us face a variety of risks to our health as we go about our day-to-day lives. Driving in cars, flying in planes, engaging in recreational activities and being exposed to environmental pollutants (air, water, food etc.) all pose varying degrees of risk.

- Some risks are simply unavoidable.

- Some we choose to accept because to do otherwise would restrict our ability to lead our lives the way we want.

- And some are risks we might decide to avoid… if we had the opportunity to make informed decisions and intelligent choices.

* * * * *

ONE OF THE GREATEST "UNKNOWN" RISKS IS.

"INDOOR AIR POLLUTION"

— THE SILENT KILLER —

Indoor air pollution is one risk that you can do something about.
Inside air can be more polluted than outside air and usually is —

In the last several years, a growing body of scientific evidence has shown that the [air in our homes] and other buildings can be and usually is, more seriously polluted than the outdoor air in even the largest and most industrialized cities **AND THIS, UNKNOWN TO MOST PEOPLE, CAUSES A VARIETY OF SERIOUS ILLNESSES, SERIOUS LONG TERM EFFECTS AND EVEN DEATH.**

An estimated 3.6 + Million deaths occur each year from **illnesses related to indoor air pollution.**

Research indicates that people spend approximately 90 percent of their time indoors… So, for many people, the risks to health may be greater due to exposure to air pollution **"indoors"** than outdoors.

Mainly — from Carbon Dioxide that is expelled from the lungs of the person or persons living in a home or an apartment — <u>especially when the doors and the windows are kept closed and sealed from outside air</u>.

[Prior to the 1970s and 80s, most people never closed their doors and windows in order to increase the efficiency of their air conditioning systems or their heating systems. They insisted on having **"Fresh Air"** in their homes]. — Mainly for health reason and for comfort — **AND… "To Have A Healthy Life." Then… A DANGEROUS CHANGE CAME ABOUT…**

—For several years now since the 1970s and '80s, it has become customary for people to close all of their doors and windows (and even seal their windows and doors) in order to increase the efficiency of their air conditioning systems and also their heating systems — WHY? To save a few pennies?

THIS IS DEFINITELY THE WRONG THING TO DO

This is completely wrong! And it is definitely jeopardizing the health of anyone and everyone living in these homes or dwelling places...

— Especially the young children —

People who spend most of their time indoors are often those most susceptible to the effects of indoor air pollution.

—Such groups include the very young, the elderly and the chronically ill, especially THE VERY YOUNG CHILDREN WHO'S LUNGS AND OTHER ORGANS ARE IN THE EARLY DEVELOPING STAGES (See article on children below).—

While pollutant levels from individual sources may not pose a significant health risk by themselves, most homes have more than one source that contributes to indoor air pollution.

There can be a serious risk from the cumulative effects of these sources and can cause a variety of illnesses and even death. Especially long term effects. *Yes... EVEN DEATH!*

Fortunately, there are steps that most people can take to both reduce the risk from existing sources and to prevent new problems from occurring.

Sources of indoor air pollution...
This causes the...
"Sick Building Syndrome."

FUNGUS and MYCROTOXINS —
Important: See report on page 44
Carbon Dioxide gas from second hand air (exhaled air)
and other gases.
Carbon Monoxide gas.

Unless they are buildings with special mechanical means
of ventilation, homes that are weather-ized (designed
and constructed **"erroneously"** to minimize the amount
of outdoor air that can "leak" into and out of the home),
will have higher pollutant levels than most other homes.
However, because some weather conditions can drastically
reduce the amount of outdoor air that enters a home,
pollutants can build up even in homes that are normally
considered "leaky"... so **ventilation is a must**.

What you need to know about pollution in your home.
Radon Gas
Mold and Mildew
Toxic Gas given off by Carpets and other building
materials
Dust Mites, Viruses, Fungi andMycrotoxins

LACK OF VENTILATION — The main source and the
greatest cause for pollution in the home is stale air and
lack of adequate supplies of oxygen.

(LACK OF VENTILATION prevents stale [polluted] air

from being purged from the home or building and seriously limits the "air exchange rate"). **And… this is the air that we breath all day long and at night. This air is lacking in the proper amount of oxygen to maintain good health.**

— New air is essential and is a MUST —

The air that is kept contained in a home or building (with no ventilation) contains many harmful pollutants including **"THE SILENT KILLERS"… CARBON DIOXIDE and CARBON MONOXIDE. Both are silent killers! AND — ONE OF THE GREATEST CAUSES FOR DISEASES AND MANY ILLNESSES: FUNGI (MANY DIFFERENT TYPES OF FUNGUS)**

DO YOU WANT YOUR YOUNG CHILDREN AND OTHER LOVED ONES TO SUFFER THE MANY CONSEQUENCES OF THIS UNFORTUNATE (AND UN-KNOWN) HAZARDOUS CONDITION? I'M SURE YOU DON'T. THEN YOU NEED TO DO SOMETHING ABOUT IT, RIGHT? THERE IS A "FREE" CURE! AND… A SIMPLE CURE! READ ON…

Amount of ventilation?

If too much indoor air (stale air) exits a home then too little outdoor air (oxygenated air) enters the home, this restricts the air exchange rate and limits the amount of oxygen that we breath, also… pollutants can accumulate to levels that can pose serious health problems. As little as 4% of carbon dioxide in a room can be deadly. (A little known fact to most people)

Outdoor air enters and leaves a house by infiltration, natural ventilation and mechanical ventilation.

In a process known as infiltration, outdoor air flows into the house through openings, joints and cracks in walls, floors and ceilings, and around windows and doors "if they are not sealed."

In natural ventilation, air moves through "opened" windows (and doors) and by wind. (Preferred method)

Finally, there are a number of mechanical ventilation devices, from outdoor-vented fans that intermittently remove air from single rooms, such as bathrooms and kitchens, to air-handling systems that use fans and duct work to continuously remove indoor air and distribute filtered and conditioned outdoor air to strategic points throughout the house. Simple ventilation can eliminate these costly methods.

THE FREE CURE

Increasing inside ventilation

YES — IT'S AS SIMPLE AS THAT! READ THIS!

The rate at which outdoor air replaces indoor air is described as the **"Air Exchange Rate."**

When there is little infiltration, natural ventilation or mechanical ventilation, the air exchange rate is low and POISONOUS POLLUTANT LEVELS CAN AND DO INCREASE.

The correct approach to lowering the concentration of indoor air pollutants in your home and to maximize the "Air Exchange Rate" is to INCREASE THE AMOUNT OF INDOOR AIR GOING OUT AND INCREASE THE AMOUNT OF OUTDOOR AIR COMING IN.

THIS IS VERY IMPORTANT!

This can be done by mechanical means (exhaust fans) or simply "opening windows" in each room of the home or building and keeping the air conditioning system running. This goes against what most people have been taught but **— IT IS TRUE!**

Many people complain that leaving doors or windows open puts a strain on their air conditioning units? Is this true? **No it is not true!**

AIR CONDITIONING: See details at the end of article. Many people believe the **"popular myth"** that opening doors or windows has a harmful effect or negative effect on their air conditioners and this definitely is a false belief (Originated with rumors and false reasonings).

Contrary to what most people think, because of false and misleading rumors (hearsay), leaving doors and windows open has little effect, if any, on your air conditioning system. (At worst, it could raise your electric bill a few pennies a month or a couple a bucks a month) This will be explained in detail and proven with the facts from air conditioning experts later in this article.

WHAT IS A MYTH

[**MYTH** — popular belief based on an untrue or false custom or un-factual traditional belief *(rumor) passed on from one generation to the next usually by family members (well meaning parents, relatives, friends and neighbors) and the Media.

YOUR LIFE or YOUR "AIR CONDITIONER?"

(Should you be concerned about your "Air Conditioner," or should you rather be concerned about the health, well being and comfort of your loved ones, especially your young children?)

Most home heating and cooling systems, including forced-air heating systems, do not mechanically bring fresh air into the home.

They simply recirculate the old stale exhaled air (Second Hand Air) and polluted air while heating or cooling the polluted air and then blowing it back into the rooms where it came from. (Almost as harmful as <u>second hand smoke</u> from cigarettes)

Opening windows and doors, operating window or attic fans when the weather permits, or running a window air conditioner with the vent control open **INCREASES THE OUTDOOR VENTING and THE AIR EXCHANGE RATE which is all important.**

NEXT — DEADLY MIS-INFORMATION

There exists a dichotomy between the "Energy Conservists" and "The Health Community" and it has been and still is <u>misleading most of the population</u> in this country and also in many other countries around the world as well.

PEOPLE ARE DYING A SLOW DEATH AND NOT EVEN BEING AWARE OF IT nor are they being told about this and/or the true facts. <u>THEY ARE NOT EVEN BEING WARNED</u>!

Virtually all of the air conditioning companies stress closing doors and windows and sealing leaks and cracks in a home to conserve electricity. (This dangerous advice has even been shown on TV and advised as "the proper thing to do") Even though this is true for conserving energy, they fail to explain (or consider) the negative and dangerous effects that this poses on the health of the people in these homes. (their own customers)

While this erroneous advise has a very detrimental effect on the way that we look on the situation, we are never told that this way of conserving electricity puts us in great danger health-wise. Eliminating the ventilation in our homes is one of the "<u>worse things and most dangerous things</u>" that we can do for our health and the health of our loved ones. **WE NEED FRESH AIR... PERIOD!**

On the Doug Kauffman show (The "KNOW THE CAUSE" show) Mr. Kauffman had a segment on "Indoor Air Pollution" and he went on to make the following claims: He stated that in the Jewish children's hospital in Denver Colorado the percentage rate of children with asthma went from 3+% in the 1980's to over 9% in 2002 and — possibly over 10% by2006. The main cause for these devastating results is thought to be mainly caused from Indoor Air Pollution — KEEPING DOORS AND WINDOWS CLOSED AND SEALED (WEATHER-IZED). AND — failing to use other measures to clean the air in our homes, businesses and mainly in our SCHOOLS.

AND — From the Doug Kauffman website:

SCIENCE, FUNGUS AND FUNGI

"A week doesn't go by that we don't find (often with your help!) yet another medical or societal reference to fungi causing human misery.

In September 1999, Johns Hopkins medical researchers confirmed that virtually all chronic sinus infections were due to fungus.

Not all findings are that solid. As a matter of fact, few are. Rather, scientists seem confused and startled at their own discoveries with regard to fungus. Fungus makes poisonous byproducts called mycotoxins. Antibiotics are one class of mycotoxins. Without this knowledge, however, many questions are raised when researchers stumble onto this seemingly elementary fact. Recently, **researchers have discovered that antibiotics are contributing to everything from 2nd heart attacks to breast cancer.** It is our hope that someday when discoveries like these are made, logic will supercede confusion."

* * * * *

Local bathroom or kitchen fans that exhaust outdoors remove contaminants directly from the room where the fan is located and also increase the outdoor air venting and the air exchange rate. As stated earlier, the air exchange rate is most important. But, this does not help the rest of the home. Proper ventilation is the answer.

Have you ever heard a person who lives in the country or up in the mountains say:

"Boy"... "Smell that nice fresh air"
Or...
"boy 'o boy"... "this nice fresh air
is sure good for me,"

TRUER WORDS WERE NEVER SPOKEN!

Fresh air helps purge our bodies of many of the toxic elements that we breath in and out every day, especially... carbon monoxide gas and carbon dioxide gas which are both silent killers.

These two gases, which are both silent killers... exist in every house and apartment that has poor ventilation or no ventilation.

This is very dangerous and very harmful to everyone who spends time in this environment especially the very young and the elderly.

* * * * *

See more articles like this one at: www.Newstarget.com

THE MYTH THAT KILLS THAT NOBODY TELLS US ABOUT

Original news summary:
http://my.webmd.com/content/article/93/102518.htm?
lastselectedguid=%7B5FE84E90-BC77-4056-A91C-
9531713CA348%7D
Type into the search box: "Indoor Air Pollution" and you
will see several articles about "Indoor Air Pollution."

POLLUTED AIR HARMFUL TO LUNG DEVELOPMENT IN YOUNG CHILDREN

Children who live in areas with THE POOREST AIR QUALITY are FIVE TIMES as likely to have lung development problems as those breathing cleaner air, according to findings from the largest and longest study ever published on the effect of air pollution on the health of kids and adolescents.

The study, funded in part by the National Institute of Environmental Health Sciences, followed 1,759 children living in 12 Southern California communities from age 10 to age 18.

THE LONG TERM EFFECTS FROM INDOOR AIR POLLUTION CAN BE DEVASTATING TO CHILDREN.

Lung function was tested annually, and researchers reported that children living in communities with the most air pollution were far more likely to have **"low forced expiratory volume"** - a test that provides information on the forcefulness of a person's breathing.

Abnormal results indicate changes in the function of the lung and/or lung disease.

The findings are reported in the Sept. 9 issue of The New England Journal of Medicine.

"Our study shows [significant deficits] in lung development associated with pollution exposure among kids in their late teens," says lead researcher Jim Gauderman, PhD, of the University of Southern California Keck School of Medicine.

These deficits are likely to be carried into adult life and could <u>translate into an increased risk for disease and death</u>."

STUDIES HAVE LONG LINKED AIR POLLUTION TO COMPROMISED LUNG FUNCTION IN YOUNG CHILDREN AND ADULTS, AND MORE RECENT RESEARCH SUGGESTS THAT LIVING IN A COMMUNITY WITH POOR AIR QUALITY <u>INCREASES THE RISK OF ASTHMA, EMPHYSEMA AND MANY OTHER DISEASES INCLUDING HEART ATTACK AND ALSO DEATH FROM HEART DISEASE</u>.

Lungs typically grow to full capacity **<u>during the teen years</u>**, and then lung function gradually declines throughout adulthood by about 1% per year after age 20.

HEALTH EFFECTS OF INDOOR POLLUTANTS ON — CHILDREN — AND ON ADULTS

Health effects from indoor air pollutants **may be experienced soon after exposure or, possibly, <u>years later</u> especially with young children.**

Immediate effects may show up after a single exposure or repeated exposure. These can include shortness of breath and/or labored breathing, fatigue, drowsiness, irritation of the eyes, nose and throat, headaches and occasional slight dizziness. Such immediate effects are usually short-term and treat-able.

Sometimes the treatment is simply eliminating the person's exposure to the source of the pollution if it can be identified. Symptoms of some diseases, including **asthma, hyper-sensitivity pneumonitis and humidifier fever**, may show up soon after exposure to some indoor air pollutants.

The likelihood of immediate reactions to indoor air pollutants depends on several factors. Age and pre-existing medical conditions are two important influences. In other cases, whether a person reacts to a pollutant depends on individual sensitivity, which varies tremendously from person to person.

Some people can become sensitized to biological pollutants after repeated exposures, and it appears that some people can become sensitized to chemical pollutants as well.

Certain immediate effects are similar to those from colds or other viral diseases, so it is often difficult to determine if the symptoms are a result of exposure to indoor air pollution. For this reason, it is important to pay attention to the time and place the symptoms occur. If the symptoms fade or go away when a person is away from the home and return when the person returns, an effort should be made to identify indoor air sources that may be possible causes. Some effects may be made worse by a hazardous supply of indoor air or from the heating, cooling or humidity conditions prevalent in the home.

Other health effects may show up either **years after exposure has occurred or only after long or repeated periods of exposure**. These effects, which include some respiratory diseases, heart disease and cancer, can be severely debilitating or fatal.

Pollutants and Tobacco smoke are thought to be the main causes of emphysema because these pollutants cause the release of chemicals within the air sacs of the lung that damage the walls of the air sacs. When chemicals are released, a chemical imbalance occurs. There are many different reasons this chemical imbalance occurs. Smoking causes the imbalance as well as exposure to air pollution, and irritating fumes and also dusts on the job.

It is prudent to try to improve the indoor air quality in your home even if symptoms are not noticeable.

Usually the most effective way to improve indoor air quality is to provide proper ventilation throughout the residence and eliminate individual sources of pollution or to reduce their emissions. Some sources, like those that contain asbestos, can be sealed or enclosed. Others, like gas stoves, can be adjusted to decrease the amount of emissions.

AIR CONDITIONING:

Because they are taught erroneously, most people think, that leaving doors and windows open puts a strain on their air conditioner. This is not true.

"__The air conditioner does not know if your doors are open or closed__." Your air conditioner runs just about the same whether your doors and windows are open or closed. Maybe it will run a little more often, in extreme cases, if the weather is very hot BUT . . THIS IS NOT REASON ENOUGH TO SACRIFICE YOUR HEALTH AND/OR YOUR COMFORT. When you are paying $90 to $150 or more a month on your electric bill, what is the big deal of saving a few pennies or even a few ($2-3) dollars and cause yourself __to be uncomfortable by not allowing your air conditioner to do it's job effectively__? If you have to pay the 100 or 150 dollars or more anyway, why not pay the very small amount of 2 or 3 dollars more to be comfortable. __It is poor logic to do otherwise__.

The same applies with lights and also refrigerators. AND... open windows.

Example:
Take this case for instance. The apartment had Slat "Louvered Windows" that were "__designed to allow__" fresh air in without opening the door and leaving the door open. The window is about 2 feet wide by 4 feet tall and has slats (Louvers) that are about 2 feet long and

3 inches wide and they are mounted horizontally in the window. They have a crank that is used to crank open the slats for ventilation.

In this case example; the resident had these "Louvered Windows" in the back door of the apartment. Some prior resident or the management had the glass "Slats" sealed with silicone cement? Does this not defeat the purpose? Why would anyone do this and go to the expense to have this done especially when it has a detrimental effect on their health? I will tell you why!

They — like so many people have been brain washed (Programmed) into thinking that they are saving money on their electric bill when in fact they are not saving any money at all (Or possibly an amount so small that it is really insignificant)

Example:
Electric Bill @ $60 to $100 month = $2.00 to $2.50 day. This amounts to **$.08** to **$.10** hour. This amounts to less than **.0015¢ a minute**. So for three minutes the cost amounts to about **$.0045 cent <u>without any savings for closing doors or windows</u>**. Now if you open a door or window for three minutes, the extra cost can only be a small percentage of the normal $.0045 cent cost for the three minutes.

Add this to your normal $2.00 a day cost and you have a total cost of about $2.0045. **[$2.00+ .0045= $2.0045].**

Even if you do this 10 times a day or more, the total increased cost for the day would still only be about $.045 or a little more. (A small part of a penny?) So the increase in cost for leaving a door or window open for a few minutes is really **negligible**.

When doors and windows are open it simply takes a little longer initially, to get the area to the desired temperature. Then it usually goes on and off at approximately the same rate as it did before the doors and windows were opened. The off cycle may be a little shorter in some extreme cases. The difference is very little and insignificant in most cases. As stated earlier, it could possibly add a few pennies or even a few dollars to your monthly electric bill, or in some instances, nothing at all. **Is it worth a few dollars to protect your health and the health and well being of your loved ones (your sons and daughters) and still have the comfort of air conditioning? That pertains to both Heating and Cooling.**

There is also a good reason to have air conditioning running while doors and windows are open and it is this... "**CONVECTION.**" When the air unit is on, it helps the air circulate and vent properly. Warm air rises and cool air falls. So... when the air unit is on, this causes the convection air to transfer and circulate properly so that the air exchange rate maintains the right amount of oxygen while at the same time venting the stale (EXHALED AIR) and polluted air to the outside and causing fresh air to enter your home. This is necessary for good health.
re: RJS

* * * * *

"TO BE SUCCESSFUL A PERSON MUST DO THE OPPOSITE OF WHAT THE MASSES THEMSELVES DO"

AND…

"The fool hates to be corrected by his father, but a wise son… listens to advice." AND…

"A fool hates to be corrected, but a wise person listens to advice, INVESTIGATES THE FACTS AND MAKES HIS OR HER OWN INFORMED DECISIONS." ALSO…"A fool learns from hearsay without ever investigating the true facts"…

"but a wise person does his or her own research to safeguard the truth."

SECOND HAND SMOKE
and
SECOND HAND AIR?

We hear a lot about SECOND HAND SMOKE don't we? BUT… Do we hear anything about SECOND HAND AIR? NO… WHY NOT? IT'S JUST AS BAD, POSSIBLY <u>WORSE</u>!

Second hand air (the air exhaled from persons in the home) contains many poisonous gases that are oderless, tasteless and can't be seen. Only with special test equipment.

Why don't we ever hear about this most dangerous pollutant? People are dying from this and no one tells us about it! THIS SHOULD BE A CRIME! We are erroneously taught to keep all the doors and windows closed tight. THIS IS WRONG! And PEOPLE SHOULD BE TAUGHT THE TRUTH

— BEFORE IT'S TOO LATE! —

Even the doctors fail to tell us about this most destructive situation. When a senior citizen goes to a doctor, one of the first questions he is asked is this: "Do you suffer labored breathing?" Most of the senior patients that are asked this — DO HAVE A PROBLEM WITH "LABORED BREATHING."

WHAT THEY ARE NOT TOLD IS THIS: WHEN THESE SENIORS (and others) SIT AROUND ALL DAY LONG AND ALL NIGHT LONG WITH ALL OF THEIR WINDOWS AND DOORS SHUT, THEY AUTOMATICALLY BREATH IN "SECOND HAND AIR," "POLLUTED AIR" (Possibly as bad as Second hand Smoke) AND IF ANYONE ELSE LIVES WITH THEM, THEY BREATH THE "EXHALED AIR" FROM OTHERS WHICH IS ALSO CONTAMINATED WITH POISONOUS GASES...

"THE SILENT KILLERS."

THEY ARE ALMOST NEVER TOLD ABOUT THE NEED FOR VENTILATION IN THEIR HOMES OR APARTMENTS.

THIS IS WHY PEOPLE ARE SLOWLY and UNKNOWINGLY "KILLING THEMSELVES" AND/OR MAKING THEMSELVES SERIOUSLY ILL WITH A VARIETY OF ILLNESSES.

The air conditioning companies are well meaning when they tell us to close our windows and doors but they fail to realize or for some reason fail to tell us the dangerous effect that this has on our health and the possible... endangerment to our lives and the lives and health of our children and other loved ones.

**IT'S TIME TO WAKE UP! WAKE UP AND SMELL THE FRESH AIR —
BEFORE IT'S TOO LATE!
GET EDUCATED! INVESTIGATE!**

QUIT LISTENING TO THE WRONG PEOPLE!

RADON GAS: (ALSO PAGES ON SECOND ONLY TO SMOKING)
THE GREATEST EXPOSURE TO RADON COMES . . IN THE HOME!
"OVERALL REDUCING OF RADON EXPOSURE IS AN IMPORTANT CONTRIBUTION TO THE GOAL OF GOOD QUALITY INDOOR AIR."**

VENTILATION HELPS REMOVE RADON GAS ALONG WITH OTHER AIR POLLUTANTS FROM YOUR HOME.

— WORLD HEALTH ORGANIZATION —

http://www.who.int/mediacentre/news/notes/2005/np15/en/index.html

Formaldehyde comes from a variety of building materials and new furnishings in the home.
http://www.information-engineer.com/kids/iaq.htm
http://www.doh.wa.gov/ehp/ts/IAQ/IAQPrimer.HTM

At high concentrations, most of the absorbed methylene chloride is exhaled unchanged. The remainder is metabolized to carbon monoxide, carbon dioxide, and inorganic chloride.
http://www.frankmckinnon.com/dichloromethane.htm

OTHER GASES SUCH AS: methylene chloride AND MORE (Even VOCs from your printer)
http://www.epa.gov/iaq/schools/tfs/guidee. html#Carbon%20Dioxide Each one of these sources listed here recommend **VENTILATION TO OUTSIDE AIR. (FRESH AIR — [OXYGENATED AIR])**

Have you seen the latest TV Commercials about their **"xxxx Air Purifiers"**? They make the following similar claims:

THE "EPA" CLAIMS THAT AMONG THE TOP 5 ENVIRONMENTAL RISKS IS "INDOOR AIR POLLUTION"! ETC., ETC., ETC..

COMPANIES TELL YOU ABOUT INDOOR AIR POLLUTION- THIS IS TRUE... BUT, DO THEY MENTION ANYTHING ABOUT VENTILATION AND

"AIR-RATE-EXCHANGE"? NO!

DO THEY MENTION THE HEALTH HAZARDS? NO!

THEY JUST WANT TO SELL YOU A PRODUCT!

WE WANT YOU TO HAVE THE TRUTH SO THAT YOU CAN PROTECT YOURSELF, YOUR CHILDREN AND YOUR OTHER LOVED ONES

IT'S TIME FOR PEOPLE TO WAKE UP!

WAKE UP AND SMELL THE COFFEE AND... "THE FRESH AIR" BEFORE IT'S TOO LATE! GET EDUCATED!

QUIT LISTENING TO THE WRONG PEOPLE!

**There are an estimated 3,800 lung cancer deaths per year in Pennsylvania alone... due to residential radon exposure.

(No one ever tells us about this do they?)

Have you ever checked your house or living quarters for radon? A kit costs about ten bucks on the Internet.

* * * * *

Cross Ventilation Air Conditioning and Thermostats Cross ventilation is key

Air needs to flow throughout the house or apartment, so make sure you open windows on both sides. If you have air conditioning, make sure the cooler air can circulate freely.

Window fans work best when blowing air out, so put your fan on the sunny side of the apartment and let it expel the hot air while pulling cool air from open windows on the shady side.

Most people have a misunderstanding about thermostats and how AC works.

Most think that if they set it a little higher (warmer) it will save money on the electric bill. Not True!

Most air conditioner thermostats are set too high (Warmer)……….. Often its operation is misunderstood. Your air conditioner runs no faster, no longer and no harder at a lower (cooler) setting, it only runs a bit longer the first time it runs.

After it reaches a certain pre-set temperature, it then runs approximately the same length of time that it would run to maintain the temperature at either a higher or lower temperature. It only takes a certain amount of time to cool the temp from say 82 degrees down to 80 degrees. It also takes the same amount of time to cool the temp down from say 79 degrees down to 78 or 76 degrees which is the average recommended for most people. It doesn't run any longer or harder at either setting. Except when the temp gets up to 100 degrees to 110 degrees or more. Then of course it will take a little longer to cool the residence

The only thing that makes it run longer is the outside temperature. When the outside temperature rises to a higher temperature your AC has to run longer at either setting because it takes longer to cool a room when it is hotter outside. Especially when the temp gets up to 100 degrees to 110 degrees or more.

CONCLUSION:

Changing the temperature setting on your thermostat (Unless it is set so that the AC doesn't come on at all) won't save any substantial amount of money on your electric bill. There is only one way to lower the cost and that is to turn off the AC once in awhile but you must then suffer the consequences.

The recommended summer setting is 76 degrees. Set it 2 to 5 degrees higher when you're away in the day or turn it off while you are away. Recent research reveals that home cooling costs increase $30 dollars month for each 30 degree rise in the outside air temperature.

The thermostat is miscalibrated... and so is the thermometer on the thermostat faceplate. The system cools lower or higher than the temperature **selected by the resident**.

For example, the thermostat might be set on 78 degrees, but an accurate thermometer shows that it's actually cooling to only 82 or 83 degrees.

This is an extremely common situation – They have been found thermostats as much as — **10 degrees off**.

The simplest solution is to rest an accurate thermometer on top of the thermostat, find out how much it's off, and compensate accordingly when you set the desired indoor temperature. *(By the way, if you'd like to receive a simple card-sized thermometer that's perfect for this kind of testing, call Energy Services at 891-0020).*

LIGHTS

All the lights in the house are on.......... or nearly all.

In most homes lighting only accounts for about 6% of the electric cost.

If you have one 75 watt light on for example, the cost (at $.008 per kilowatt hour) is less than a penny for one hour. — $.008

Although, it is prudent to conserve, it is not logical to run around telling everyone to turn off the LIGHTS all the time. You are lucky if you save 4-5 cents a day and cause a lot of confusion for family members and guests and also irritate many… "**JUST TO SAVE A FEW PENNIES**"?

When your electric bill averages $75 to $100 sometimes even $150 dollars, it doesn't make sense to worry about saving a few pennies or even a few dollars by weather-izing your home, sealing windows and doors and worrying about someone keeping a door open too long. What most people don't realize is that they are doing all this worrying for nothing and I will explain.

People think for two reasons that they can save a ton of money on their hugh electric bills. Well they can't! And I will tell you why.

First of all a lot of "Well Meaning" companies out there (Mostly Air Conditioning Companies) tell us how to conserve our electricity by sealing windows and doors. Weather-izing our homes and more. **THIS IS WRONG**! YOU WILL SEE!

While these people and their companies are correct in a technical way and they mean well they are misleading many. They never tell us about "THE SILENT KILLERS" —

"THE INDOOR AIR POLLUTION." IT'S TRUE — MILLIONS ARE DYING EVERY YEAR FROM THIS UNKNOWN KILLER.

AND IT IS RUINING THE HEALTH OF MILLIONS HERE IN THE UNITED STATES OF AMERICA AND ALSO AROUND THE WORLD!

— THIS IS NO JOKE —

* * * * *

THE SICK BUILDING SYNDROME

(We hardly ever hear about this. Most never hear)

Refer to:
http://www.doctorfungus.org/mycoses/environ/sick_
building.htm

* * * * *

The indoor environment is a creation of the modern era. Previously, buildings were notable for the extent to which they were really open to the outside air, a system that could be referred to as natural ventilation. But, technological advances have permitted us to seal buildings tightly, recirculate the air within them, and fill them with a variety of particle- and chemical-emitting materials and objects.

Complaints and anecdotes regarding illnesses produced by life inside such buildings have become commonplace. Several categories of these illnesses have been proposed.

Specific Illnesses

- Indoor transmission of standard infectious diseases such as tuberculosis or legionellosis.
- Allergic reactions to indoor allergens such as dust mites, plant products, or fungal products. .
- Irritation due to (volatile) chemicals released from the environment.
- Carbon monoxide poisoning related to recirculation of cigarette smoke or exhaust fumes.

Non-Specific Illnesses

- This is a diverse group of work-related symptoms that include irritation of the skin, mucus membranes (mouth, nose, throat), headache, fatigue, and difficulty concentrating.
- A variety of factors have been associated with increased rates of these complaints: younger age, female sex, cigarette smoking, type of work (e.g., working near a photocopier), level of office crowding, presence of carpets, and type/volume of ventilation.
- Environmental mycology covers issues in facilities that range from industrial settings where fungi impact manufacturing processes, to **"home and work environments" and "hospitals"** where human health may be an issue. There currently is extensive interest in understanding the health implications of fungi in **indoor environments**. Questions related to these issues are among the most common types of questions received by "DoctorFungus." The key current challenges in this area are:
- How does one detect and measure the presence of indoor fungi?
- What is an acceptable level of indoor fungi?
- How do we relate this information to human health problems?
- How do we control the level of fungi in our environment?

A week doesn't go by that we don't find (often with your help!) yet another medical or societal reference to fungi causing human misery. In September 1999, Johns Hopkins medical researchers confirmed that virtually all chronic sinus infections were due to fungus. Not all findings are that solid.

As a matter of fact, few are. Rather, scientists seem confused and startled at their own discoveries with regard to fungus. Fungus makes poisonous byproducts called mycotoxins. Antibiotics are one class of mycotoxins.

Without this knowledge, however, many questions are raised when researchers stumble onto this seemingly elementary fact. Recently, researchers have discovered that antibiotics are contributing to everything from 2nd heart attacks to breast cancer. It is our hope that someday when discoveries like these are made, logic will supercede confusion.

Fungi are not the Only Problem

Even though fungi are components of indoor air quality (IAQ), many other factors may contribute to indoor air quality problems.

Non-biological contaminants include asbestos, radon, tobacco smoke, pesticides, lead, and carbon monoxide. Biological contaminants include viruses, bacteria such as the aerobic actinomycetes, mites and their fecal material, insects such as moths and cockroaches, dander from people and pets, algae, and pollen may also cause problems. Indoor-related health issues might result from more than one of these potential etiologic agents having a simultaneous effect on the occupants. The EPA's The Inside Story: A Guide to Indoor Air Quality [92] is available for downloading from the EPA IAQ web site and is an outstanding review of this area.

* * * * *

CAN WE BELIEVE ALL OF THE FACTS THAT WE ARE GIVEN?

QUOTE FROM: KTRE.com

GO TO: http://www.ktre.com/Global/story.asp?S=3176982

QUOTE: "Lung cancer is the number one cancer killer of men and women in the world."
Dr. Roberts said, "There are about 180,000 cases a year in the United States."

NUMBER ONE KILLER? — IS THIS A TRUE STATEMENT OF FACT?
* * * * *

QUOTE FROM: BBC NEWS

GO TO: http://news.bbc.co.uk/1/hi/health/1015657.stm

We are told: "Cancer remains the main cause of death in both men and women, according to the Department of Health."

Between 1950 and 1999, deaths due to cancer rose from 15% to 27% in men and from 16% to 23% in women - overtaking heart disease, stroke and infectious diseases as the other major killers in England and Wales.

QUOTE: "Cancer currently kills 135,000 people a year, compared to 110,000deaths from heart disease."
Is it really The main cause of death?

HOW CAN THE ABOVE STATEMENTS BE TRUE WHEN IN FACT OVER "3.6 MILLION PEOPLE DIE... EACH YEAR" FROM INDOOR AIR POLLUTION IN THE UNITED STATES ALONE?

WHAT ABOUT IT?

WHAT ABOUT THE 3.6 MILLION THAT DIE FROM INDOOR AIR POLLUTION?
QUOTE: "3.6 MILLION PEOPLE DIE EACH YEAR FROM INDOOR AIR POLLUTION IN THE UNITED STATES ALONE."

DO YOU SEE WHAT IS BEING IGNORED?

DO YOU SEE WHAT IS BEING MISSED?

NO DOCTORS OR AGENCIES EVEN WARNS US ABOUT THIS KILLER. WHY?

WHY DOES THIS CRUCIAL ISSUE NEVER MAKE THE NEWS WHEN SO MANY ARE DYING?

JUST LOOK ON THE INTERNET — THERE IS EVIDENCE, EVIDENCE, EVIDENCE!

I am not claiming that these numbers are correct or that they are incorrect, I am just showing you that the facts often get misconstrued and lead us to believe some things that are not necessarily true.

AND... THIS MOST IMPORTANT FACT GOES UN-NOTICED OR IGNORED BY THE NEWS MEDIA and OTHERS!

The following is from: OSHA and the American Biological Safety Association (ABSA).

Poor indoor air quality is one of the most important health issues we face today.

Molds and fungi are found in virtually every environment and can be detected both indoors and outdoors year round.

The number of species of existing molds and fungi is estimated from tens of thousands to three hundred thousand or more. Molds and fungi produce and release millions of spores small enough to be air-, water-, or insect-borne. They can also produce toxic agents known as mycotoxins. Spores and mycotoxins can have negative effects on human health including allergic reactions, asthma and other respiratory problems.

This page is maintained as a product of the Alliance between OSHA and the American Biological Safety Association (ABSA).

* * * * *

The following is taken from the Internet:
http://www.aerias.org/kview.asp?spaceid=1

Where are mycotoxins found?

TO CHECK ON MYCOTOXINS IN THE HOME GO TO:
http://www.aerias.org/kview.asp?spaceid=1

THERE YOU WILL SEE A PICTURE OF A HOUSE AND YOU MAY PICK A SPICIFIC ROOM OR PART OF THE HOUSE SO THAT YOU MAY RESEARCH DIFFERENT ARTICLES, REPORTS AND/OR INFORMATION.

THIS IS WHAT YOU WILL SEE AND YOU

CAN CLICK ON DIFFERENT AREAS OF THE HOUSE TO ACCESS REPORTS ETC.

* * * * *

The following examples are about plants and animals and are used here just to show how prevalent mycotoxins are in the food and animal industry and these are also found in homes due to poor air quality.

These examples are for reference only.

— FUNGAL DISEASES —

Fungal diseases are common place in plants and animals.

In such diseases, the fungi are actively growing on and invading the body of their hosts.

There is another means by which fungi can cause harm without invading our bodies. When fungi grow on a living organism or on stored food material that we consume, they may produce harmful metabolites that diffuses into their food. It is believed that fungi evolved these metabolites as a means of protecting their food supply by preventing other organisms from eating it.

44

These metabolites are referred to as **mycotoxins**, which literally means "fungus poisons". Fungi that produce mycotoxins do not have to be present to do harm.

If a fungus was growing in, say a grain storage silo, the environment may have become unsuitable for the fungus and it dies. Even though the fungus is no longer alive, while it was growing, if it produced a mycotoxin, it will have poisoned the grains. So for those of you who are always looking to save a little money by buying cheese that has been contaminated with a fungus and cutting out the part where the fungus is growing, perhaps this is not such a good idea.

It is possible that the fungus growing on your cheese has produced a mycotoxin that has diffused throughout the cheese, even though the fungus itself has not. The effects of poisoning by mycotoxin is referred to as **mycotoxicoses**.

The knowledge that mycotoxicoses is the result of fungal actions was a relatively, recent discovery. This is understandable since illnesses in this case is due to consumption of mycotoxins that has been released by the fungus and is not directly caused by the fungus. So demonstrating this would not have been an easy task. We now know that many species of fungi produce mycotoxins, but why?

It is thought fungi have evolved production of various mycotoxins in order to prevent other fungi or animals from consuming "their" food. By secreting their mycotoxin into their food the fungus will inhibit growth of other fungi and discourage rotten or other small animals from eating their food.

45

There have been several lectures given and several studies conducted on mycotoxins.

The existence of mycotoxins was not documented until 1960. However, just as in the case of diseases, the concept that mold in your home could lead to illness in people or domestic animals was long suspected before their existence was demonstrated by science. It is a greater problem, presently than it was in the distant past.

Long ago, before there was adequate means of long term storage for perishable goods, food was normally consumed a short time after it was acquired, but as the world has becomemore industrialized and technological advanced, storage of food has become more of an issue. One our issues is mold in the home.

Food is now commonly stored for long periods of time, giving fungi a greater opportunity to contaminate our food. Before 1900, in Italy, researchers there believed consumption of moldy corn by children led to the development of illness. Some experiments, done at that time, included the isolation, and growth of the suspected fungus in pure culture, and isolation of toxic compounds from the fungus that the researchers believed to be the cause of the illness. This can also be caused by some types of mold found in many homes.

However, since the compound was not identified and was not actually isolated from the moldy corn, it could not be concluded that this compound was the cause of the illness or that the compound in question was even present on the moldy corn. Nevertheless, it appeared that there was a correlation between the illness and consumption of moldy corn, but this did not eliminate the possibility that it was the fungus, itself, that caused the disease, which most people believed to be the case. It was also possible that there were other reasons for the illnesses that were observed.

A study conducted in 1957 showed an extensive outbreak of moldy corn disease in the southeastern United States in the early 1950's where hundreds of wild pigs foraging in cultivated corn fields became ill, and many died. Teams of veterinarians and mycologists collaborated to determine the cause of the deaths of these pigs. They isolated a number of different fungi from the moldy corn and inoculated each fungus on moist corn that had been sterilized and then fed them to pigs.

The consumption of corn inoculated with *Aspergillus flavus* caused outward signs and inward lesions found in other cases of the so-called moldy corn disease. However, since there was no toxin(s) isolated, there was little attention paid to the article since it still seemed like old news, i.e. domestic animals poisoned by eating moldy corn.

THESE ARE JUST EXAMPLES OF WHAT DIFFERENT MOLDS CAN DO

It would not be until 1960, when approximately 100,000 turkeys and a lesser number of other domestic birds died in England, causing losses of approximately several hundred thousand dollars, before the first mycotoxin was isolated and identified.

This did not happen immediately. Initially, the disease was thought to be caused by a virus and the syndrome was named "**turkey-X disease.**" The "X" here indicated that the cause of the disease was unknown. However, with a great deal of detective work, on the parts of the researchers, soon the cause of the disease was traced to feed that was produced by Oil Cake Mills, Ltd. (research always seems to get done more quickly and receive more priority when loss of large sums of money is involved).

The oil cake feed was composed mostly of peanuts. However, it seemed unlikely that the peanut meal itself was toxic, since peanut meal had long been used as a feed ingredient and was known to be an excellent source of protein. Thus, it was reasoned that something must have been added to the peanut meal to make it toxic, and one possibility that was investigated was that peanuts had been made toxic by "fungi" growing in them.

From their isolations, the investigators identified *Aspergillus flavus*, the same fungus that was isolated by Burnside and his research teams. The isolated fungus was again inoculated into the feed and fed to the turkeys. Shortly after feeding, the turkeys died with external signs and internal lesions identical to those observed in the birds that had previously died in the field.

Unlike Burnside, however, chemists were also employed in this investigation, and they were able to isolate and identify the toxin from the oil cake feed.

The mycotoxin isolated was named **aflatoxin**, the "a" from *Aspergillus* and "fla" from *flavus*. Feeding test of food containing aflatoxin, with various laboratory animals, demonstrated that to varying degrees, all animals tested were sensitive to aflatoxin. Even consumption of extremely small amounts of aflatoxin damaged various internal organs and could induce development of cancer to the liver.

This was of great concern among the nutritionists and those concerned with problems of pubic health, the Food and Drug Administration Etc..
There was great concern domestically since peanuts and peanut products were and still are of economic importance. It was also of international significance since peanuts at that time were being lauded as an excellent source of protein for developing countries by United Nations International Children's Emergency Fund and other such organizations. Deficiency in protein often results in "kwashiorkor."

Kwashiorkor (kwa´shê-ôr´kôr´), protein deficiency disorder of children, prevalent in overpopulated parts of the world where the diet consists mainly of starchy vegetables, particularly Africa, Central and South America, and S Asia. Such a diet is deficient in certain amino acids, which make up proteins vital for growth.

Depending on the extent and duration of the deficiency manifestations include skin changes, edema, severely bloated abdomen, diarrhea, and generally retarded development.

Other characteristics include anemia, depigmentation of the skin, and loss of hair or change in hair color…

Usually occurring in children shortly after weaning Peanut products were developed in various forms, especially in tropical and subtropical countries for general distribution.

Were these people now exchanging kwashiorkor for potential risk of liver damage and cancer from consuming aflatoxins?

There was a great deal at stake which provided the need to act on this matter immediately.

In the United States as soon as awareness of aflatoxins surfaced in the 1960's programs were established by peanut growers to reduce the possibility of aflatoxin occurring in edible peanuts and peanut products.

The Fungus

Aspergillus flavus is actually not a single species, but a "species complex," made up of eleven species that are known to occur in many kinds of plant materials, including stored grains. One of the species in the complex *A.oryzae* has long been used in the Orient to prepare various kinds of food products such as sake, tofu and soy sauce which in turn is used in the United States. Were aflatoxins present in these products as well?

This was a question that needed to be answered. Research began to take place at a rapid pace and continues to do so. The number of papers published that have to do with aflatoxins number in the hundreds annually.

This may sound strange but in some cultures, fungi are encouraged to grow on certain foods in order to give them the desired taste.

The Bantu tribes in Africa prefer the sour flavor of partly

spoiled corn to that of fresh corn and fungus is purposely allowed to grow on the corn for this reason (Christensen, 1975). However, this may only be a coincident, ***but they also have a very high incident of primary liver cancer***.

How much aflatoxin is too much?

In 1972 for over a period of several years 100 different samples of black pepper from all over the world were examined. In a few of these cultures, of these samples the number of fungus colonies in whole or ground black pepper averaged 52,000 per gram/black pepper and the upper range was over half a million per gram. These colonies were mostly of *A.flavus*, *A.ochraceus* and *A.versicolor*.

All three species are known to be aflatoxin producers. Some samples of ground pepper were caked lightly with fungus mycelium when first opened in the laboratory and with time, a number of these became solidly caked with mycelium.

How heavily contaminated is 52,000 to 500,000 colonies of fungi, per gram? Lets make a comparison for what is acceptable levels of fungal colonies isolated in other food products at the time the results were published.

Wheat for example that is intended for milling into flour seldom contains less than a few thousand colonies of fungi per gram of grain. If barley has as many as 10,000 colonies of the same kind of fungi per gram as in black pepper it would be rejected for malting in beer making. If breakfast cereals or bread were as contaminated as black peppers they would have so musty an odor and taste that they would not be fit to eat. Apparently, the natural spicy odor and flavor of black as well as white pepper are potent enough to conceal the taste and odor of these fungi. This is also true with many other spices.

What about the processed food prepared with *A.flavus*?

At least in the commercial strains that have been utilized to prepare food in the United States the strains that have been tested have not been found to produce aflatoxins.

However, where these products are prepared in a household or village industry and the fungus is just carried from one batch to the next, wild strains capable of producing aflatoxin may contaminate them. In an investigation in the Philippines, not a single sample was found that was free of aflatoxin. In such communities probably everyone was suffering to some extent from chronic aflatoxin poisoning.

What does this have to do with Indoor Air Pollution?

Plenty! This just shows a picture of what the fungi are all about and these are in most homes around the country and around the world.

Mycotoxins in Other Species of *Aspergillus*, *Penicillium* and *Fusarium*

Aspergillus ochraceus and ochratoxin

Aspergillus ochraceus is also a species complex and consist of nine species. These species are common in soil, decaying vegetation and in stored seeds and grains undergoing microbial deterioration. However, this fungus is seldom isolated from more than a small percentage of seeds or grains that are undergoing microbiological deterioration in storage because it is evidently not a good competitor as is also the case with *A.flavus*.

This is a general rule but at the University of Minnesota *A.ochraceus* sometimes has been isolated from 40% or more of surface-disinfected kernels of corns from bins in which deterioration was in progress. It has also been the major organism in some lots of whole black pepper. Also, samples of macaroni and spaghetti were found to be heavily invaded by this species.

Production of ochratoxin, by *A.ochraceus*, was first described in South Africa by Theron, *et al.* (1966), where it was isolated along with a number of other fungi. In experiments done with this isolate the LD50 (the single dose that will kill 50 percent of the individual animals tested) of ochratoxin for rats is 22mg/kg (= 22 milligrams of the toxin per kilogram of body weight of the rat), but a lesser amount will result in severe liver damage. A single dose of 12.5 mg/kg (=12.5 milligrams of the toxin per kilogram of body weight of the rat) was administered to pregnant rats on the tenth day of gestation, and of the 88 fetuses involved, 72, or 81.8% died or were resorbed. Ducklings seem to be equally sensitive to ochratoxin as they are to aflatoxin.

Another fungus, *Penicillium viridicatum*, can also produce ochratoxin, and is relatively common in stored corn and is a more common producer of ochratoxin than *A.ochraceus*.

Aspergillus versicolor and sterigmatocystin

This species is another storage fungus.

However it is never found as the only fungus or as the predominating fungus in deteriorating cereals. Normally by the time a grain sample has become very moldy *A.versicolor* along with other *Aspergillus* species and usually other filamentous fungi and yeasts as well. Some of the black pepper mentioned earlier, as being decayed by fungi, was very heavily invaded by *A.versicolor*, but not by this fungus exclusively.

One rather interesting case concerning this species took place on germinating barley in a malthouse in Scotland. The growth of *A.versicolor* was so luxuriant on the germinating barley and produced so many spores that the workers who turned the malts with shovels could not see one another because of the spore-filled air. The owners and managers of the malthouse hired a mycologist to determine how the fungus was getting in. They had assumed that the contamination must have been due to the incoming barley. What the mycologist concluded was that there was a lack of sanitaryconditions in the malthouse and that everything in and around that malthouse must have been thoroughly and heavily contaminated by *A.versicolor* spores and probably a lot of other fungi as well. So when conditions were favorable when the barley was brought in, the growth of fungi grew to spectacular quantities. Can you imagine working in such an environment and having to inhale those spores?

(We have similar thing floating around in our homes especially when our windows and doors are kept closed)

This species sometimes produces sterigmatocystin, a toxic compound given the name because the fungus once was called Sterigmatocystis. The toxin is known to causelung and liver tumors in laboratory animals and has been implicated as the cause of disease in calves that have consumed feed heavily invaded by A.versicolor.

Aspergillus fumigatus and fumagillin

This particular species is known to be an animal pathogen. Infection occurs through inhalation of spores and affects the lungs.

Infection may also occur in eggs and the fetuses of cows. However it also produces a metabolic product that may be considered a toxin or an antibiotic. This species differs from the others that we have discussed in that it is said to be **thermophilic**. It is found in substrate where there are extremely high temperatures, up to 122°F (=50°C). This species is usually found on material that is in the advanced stages of decomposition in which the substrate temperature has been significantly raised by microbial decomposition.

Under the proper conditions *A.fumigatus* produces **fumagillin**.

This compound is used as an amoebicide. Used as a means to rid the body of amoebae that are human pathogens and has been used effectively in honey bees as well. The correct dosage of this compound is critical.

The Genus *Fusarium*

Species of Fusarium are widespread in nature as saprobes in decaying vegetation and as parasites on all parts of plants. Many cause diseases of economically important plants. For this reason there has been a great deal of research carried out by both plant pathologist and mycologist. However there are a number of species that produce mycotoxins. Mostly **trichothecenes** and zearalenone.

Fusarium tricinctum

The effects of the first trichothecene toxin T-2 were documented in the 1940s where it was associated with an outbreak of alimentary toxic aleukia(ATA). At its peak in 1944 the population in the Orenbury District and other districts of the then USSR suffered enormous casualties. More than 10 percent of the population was affected and many fatalities occurred.

The term *alimentary* toxic refers to the toxin being consumed in foods and *aleukia* refers to the reduced number of leucocytes or white blood cells inthe affected person. Other symptoms included bleeding from nose and throat and multiple subcutaneous hemorrhages.

The infected food in this case was millet which made up a great part of the diet of the people in the region and at times during WWII it was not uncommon to allow the millet to be left standing in the fields over winter because bad weather in the fall prevented its harvest at the proper time.

During the late winter and early spring the millet would become infected with a variety of fungi including *F.tricinctum* and when the people gathered and ate this fungus many came down with what was diagnosed as ATA. Thousands were affected and many died.

Joffe, a plant pathologist determined to be the outbreak of ATA was caused by consumption of a toxin present in the millet which had been contaminated by *F. tricinctum*. This was a remarkable conclusion since this was 20 years before aflatoxin was discovered. However, Joffe did not isolate or identify the toxin involved and as a result his work remained unknown until about 1965 when he presented a summary of his research at a symposium on mycotoxins.

The mycotoxin involved was later given the common name **T-2** and classified as one of several trichothecenes.
When fed to rats it has an LD50 of 3.8mg/kg which is lower than that of aflatoxin but still toxic enough.

Fusarium graminearum

Corn is a stable in many countries and is used as a major ingredient in preparation of food for pigs and other domestic animals. Like many other grains the kernels can be infected with fungi before and after harvest and can affect the nutritional value of corn as food or feed.

If the weather is rainy and the ears of corn are maturing in late summer and early fall *F. graminearum* may infect only a few to a third of the kernels. Whatever amount of the ear is infected all the kernels in that portion becomes heavily infected and decayed by the fungus. This fungus infected corn is unattractive to pigs, as well as other animals, and they refuse to it.

Regardless of what the composition of the rest of the feed, if it contains more than 5 percent of kernels the pigs will not eat it and weight loss will occur. They will starve rather than consume it.

The infected corn contains an emetic compound produced by the fungus and if this corn is consumed by pigs they suffer prolonged vomiting after which they sensibly refuse to eat more of the corn. The toxin involved is deoxynivalenol (DON) also known as **vomitoxin**. The isolation and identification of this toxin has occurred only within the last 25 years.

The detection of infected corn or feed is also a problem. Since we are talking about mycotoxin, here the inability to isolate the causal agent *F.graminearum*, is not evidence that the mycotoxin is absent. Long after a fungus has died off, mycotoxin secreted into the substrate will still be present.

Use of Trichothecenes as a Biological Weapon

Yellow Rain

During the mid 1970's when Vietnam was invading Laos there were stories of "yellow rain" in areas where entire villages were killed. One eye witness account of such an event was told by a refugee in Thailand. While tending his poppies outside of his village he and his family witnessed the bombing of their village by the Vietnamese in MIGS with a yellow powder that came down like yellow rain. Returning to the village he found all of the animals and most of the people were dead.

The bodies were bleeding from the nose and ears and their skin were blistered and yellowed. The few people left alive when he arrived were jerking like fish when you take them out of the water. These people also eventually died. The witness took his family away from the village but as they left they felt shortness of breath and sick to their stomach. This story is similar to other stories that were heard concerning yellow rain.

The media and scientific community gave critical examination of the yellow rain story. The analysis that demonstrated Trichothecenes were being used was initially based on a single leaf collected where one of the chemical attacks occurred. Subsequent specimens were collected later that also showed Trichothecenes were present but the ratio of trichothecenes differed where it was found and was entirely absent in some samples. In addition little fanfare was given to the over one hundred samples analyzed by the United States Army which *did not find any indication of trichothecenes.*

Trichothecenes and the Lack of Population Increase in Europe

Something very interesting concerning mycotoxins in fungi has recently come to light.

Historical demographers or the people that study populations, their distribution, density and other such vital statistics have shown that long life and good health are a recent phenomenon.

Before 1750 in England the life expectancy of a member of the British peerage, that is one who has borne of noble birth, was only 36.7 years old. A hundred years later it had risen to 58.4 years. Conditions were worse and improvement was slow among the common folks. But, between 1750 and 1850 the population of Europe almost doubled.

Before 1750 good health was a privilege of wealth and not even then did all the rich enjoy it. A commoner was often underweight, stunted, sickly and occasionally deranged. They could not even imagine the feeling of well being that we have today. There was a constant battle with death. There were great fluctuations in populations because of mortality crises. After a mortality crisis more people in a community would marry and they would marry younger and would eventually give rise to more children so that if things were normal a community would tend to produce more babies than corpses. But then pretty soon another crisis would come. A disease, famine, natural disasters, etc. and the gain in population would be wiped out.

You might not know it but cereals come from plants that are seldom free of molds and it is a theory that it was the consumption of such contaminated grains that had damaged the immune system of the population of Europe that had relied on grain as their staple and was probably largely responsible for a short life span. T-2 and related trichothecenes are known to compromise an individual's immune system. It would be a change of diet that would begin to give individuals a longer life span.

Mycological Terms

Aflatoxins: First mycotoxins discovered, in 1960, produced by *Aspergillus flavus*.

Aleukia Toxic Aleukia (ATA): Condition associated with consumption of trichothecenes mycotoxin T-2 produced by *Fusarium tricinctum*. Some symptoms of condition include low white blood cell count, multiple subcutaneous hemorrhages and bleeding from nose and throat.

Aspergillus flavus: Species complex in which first mycotoxins and aflatoxins were discovered.

Aspergillus fumigatus: Species of fungi producing mycotoxin and antibiotic fumagillin.

Fumagillin: Compound produced by *Aspergillus fumigatus*. Although classified as a mycotoxin it is also effectively used as an antibiotic for amoebic parasites in humans as well as honeybees. The dosage is very important here.

If too much is used, it can be fatal.

Fusarium graminearum: Species associated with production of mycotoxin and vomitoxin which causes pigs and other animals not to consume food when present. Pigs would initially eat food containing toxin but after a prolonged period of vomiting they refused to consume more food with toxin.

Fusarium tricinctum: Species producing trichothecenes associated with alimentary toxic aleukia (ATA). First documented in 1940's of USSR.

Kwashiorkor: Protein deficiency disorder of children in various overpopulated countries in the world.

Historians believed that the population depression that occurred in Europe before 1750 was due to consumption of moldy grains that contained mycotoxins. It was believed that such mycotoxins reduced fertility and life span of individuals and that it was not until a change in diet from grains to potatos did the situation improved. Between 1750 and 1850 the population of Europe doubled as a result of change in diet.

Mycotoxicoses: The effects of poisoning from mycotoxins.

Mycotoxins: Poisons from fungi.

T-2: Trichothecene mycotoxin produced by Fusarium tricinctum that is associated with ATA.

Vomitoxin: Name given to trichothecenes that causes pigs and other animals to refuse food containing this mycotoxin. Pig would initially eat food with toxin but after a prolonged period of vomiting the pig would refuse to eat it even when hungry.

* * * * *

While great care has been taken in the preparation of the material in this book medicine is a rapidly changing field.

As new research and experience broaden our knowledge changes in the approach to diagnosis and therapy become necessary and appropriate.

Recommendations made in this book are only recommendations based on the information provided by agencies, people, groups and organizations publishing reports and information on the Internet and other media.

The information provided here may not always apply precisely to an individual's situation. AND — consultations with a physician and other professionals should be undertaken before following any of the strategies suggested in this book and/or on our web site.

Copywrite©2006TransWorld International

SEE THE FOLLOWING FOR TYPICAL COSTS FOR ELECTRICAL APPLIANCE

FOR TYPICAL COSTS SEE FOLLOWING STATISTICS

HEALTH & BEAUTY
Curling Iron 30 w, 19¢/year
Electric Razor 14w, 3¢/year
Hair-dryer 1200 w, 2¢/15 min.
Hot Rollers 350 w, 1¢/30 min

HOME ENTERTAINMENT
CD Player 10 w, 1¢/15 hrs.
Stereo 16 w, 1¢/10 hrs.
Light Bulb 60 w, 1¢ / 15 hrs. = .06¢ hr.
1 Light Bulb - **1/15th of a penny** for **one hour**.

Television 110 w, 4¢/day = $1.20 a month
TVs consume 75% of total wattage when not in use.
VCR/DVD 25 w, 1¢/6 hrs.
Video Games 17 w, 1¢/10 hrs.
DSS Satellite Receiver 24 w, 1¢/8 hrs.

HOUSEWARES
Wall Clock 4 w, 5¢/month
Sewing Machine 175 w, 1¢/hr.
Vacuum Cleaner 1300 w, 9¢/hr.
Central Vacuum 1440 w, 10¢/hr

LAUNDRY
Iron 1008 w, 7¢/hr.
Washing Machine 512 w, 2¢/load

Clothes Dryer 5500 w, 27¢/load

Water Heater 4500 w, 94¢/day= $28.00 Month

**Kitchen Freezer - manual defrost (20 cu. ft.)
600 w, 32¢/day 32¢/day = $10.00 Month**

Can Opener 100 w, 1¢/hr.
Coffee Maker 894 w, 1¢/pot
Dishwasher 1201 w, 7¢/load
Garbage Disposal 700 w, 1¢/day
Microwave Oven 1450 w, 11¢/hr.
Mixer 127 w, 1¢/hr.
Range & Oven 12000 w,
22¢/day — **22¢/day = <u>$7.00 Month</u>**
Range & Self-Cleaning Oven 13700 w, 23¢/day
Electric Grill 1580 w,11¢/hr.
Toaster 1146 w, 1¢/4 servings
Bread-maker 675 w, 5¢/ hr.

GARAGE & GARDEN TOOLS
Garage Door Opener 800 w, 63¢/month
Hedge Trimmer 265 w, 2¢/hr.
Lawn-mower (cord-less) 40 w, 7¢/charge
20 hour battery charge = 1 hour mowing time
Lawn-mower (electric with cord) 561 w, 4¢/hr.
Weed-eater 300 w, 2¢/hr.

HOME OFFICE
Computer 450w, 3¢/hr.

* * * * *

THE BIGGEST COSTS FOR A MONTH

Water Heater 4500 w, 94¢/day= $28.00 Month

Kitchen Freezer - manual defrost (20 cu. ft.) 600 w, 32¢/day
32¢/day = $10.00 Month

Range & Oven 12000 w, 22¢/day 22¢/day = $7.00 Month

Heat and Air 100 - 200 Day $30-$60 Month

Miscellaneous 83¢/day = $25.00 - 1.50 day $25.00 - $45.00 Month

Total $100 to $150 Month

Conclusion:

The only way to save a significant amount of money on your electric bill is to turn off one or more of these high-cost appliances periodically. [And this is not practical for most people]

Closing doors and windows can only save approximately $4-$6 dollars a month which is about 13-14¢ a day. Lowering your air conditioner usage could only save about $3-$6 maybe even $10 or $15 dollars a month. Is this worth suffering the inconvenience of the lack of healthy fresh air and putting your health in danger and mainly the health of your loved ones? Or the lack of comfort by running your air conditioner or your heater at a few degrees lower just to save a few pennies? Is this small savings really logical?

Most people don't do the research. They simply listen to the wrong people and rely on hearsay (which is false info most of the time). And — Most of these people pass this faulty information on to their children and then on to more children and more children and it becomes customary.

This then becomes tradition and causes millions of deaths needlessly as do many other "false rumors."

Do you do what they do?

* * * * *

A tremendous amount of work and many hours of research went into the gathering of facts in order to produce this informative book. Many of the reports were accessed on the Internet and other sources as well.

This book with all of the reports is being provided in hopes that we can help prevent some of the dying of the uninformed public and protect the health of the many Americans — men, women and children and the men, women and children of neighbering Countries also.

* * * * *

www.ingramcontent.com/pod-product-compliance
Lightning Source LLC
Chambersburg PA
CBHW020401290526
45785CB00005B/2394

9781412089999